MW01107659

QUICK-E

CRITICAL CARE

Clinical Nursing Reference

Martin Schiavenato RN, BSN, MS

BANDIDO
BOOKS

Other fine titles available in the Quick-E Series:

Med-Surg

E.R.

Peds

Spanish Guide for Nurses

To keep abreast of changes, additions and new products, please
visit us at www.bandidobooks.com or contact us at
publish@bandidobooks.com or by postal service at:
Bandido Books | 9806 Heaton Court | Orlando, FL 32817
To order call our Toll-Free Hotline at 1-877-814-6824 PIN 1174

Essential Facts at Clinical Speed!

Happy Nursing!

Reviewers

With respect and admiration:
To all the nurses (and their families)
charged with caring for
the critically ill and injured.

M.S.

Contents

Laboratory Values

CBC

RBC	4.7-6.1 million/mm³ (♂)	Hgb	13.5-17.5 g/dl (♂)
	4.2-5.4 million/mm³ (♀)		12-16 g/dl (♀)
WBC	4300-10800 cells/mm³	Hct	40-54 % (♂)
			37-47 % (♀)
Platelets	150-350 thousand/mm³	MCV	80-94 cu microns
MCH	27-32 pg	MCHC	32-36 %

Chemistry

Na	135-148 mEq/L	K	3.5-5.0 mEq/L
Cl	98-106 mEq/L	CO_2	24-32 mEq/L
BUN	7-18 mg/dl	Uric Acid	3.0-7.0 mg/dl
Ca	8.5-10.5 mg/dl	Mg	1.3-2.1 mEq/L
Creatinine	0.7-1.3 mg/dl (♂)	Glucose	
	0.6-1.2 mg/dl (♀)	(fasting)	70-110 mg/dl
Bilirubin		Lipids	
	Direct 0-0.2 mg/dl		Cholesterol 120-220 mg/dl
	Total 0.2-1.0 mg/dl		Triglycerides 40-150 mg/dl
	Indirect Total minus Direct		
Osmolality	275-295 mOsm/kg	Anion gap	8-16 mEg/L
Amylase	50-150 U/L	Lipase	4-24 U/L
Alkaline Phosphatase (ALP)		SGPT (ALT)	10-55 U/L (♂)
	13-39 U/L (adults)		7-30 U/L (♀)

"Here is the test to find whether your mission on earth is finished.
If you're alive, it isn't."

Richard Bach

Sedimentation Rate

Wintrobe	0-9 mm per hour (♂)	*Westergren* 1-13 mm per hour (♂)
	0-20 mm per hour (♀)	1-20 mm per hour (♀)

Coagulation

PT	10-14 sec	PTT	30-45 sec
APTT	16-25 sec	ACT	92-128 sec
FSP	<10 mcg/dl	Platelets	150-350 thousand/mm³

INR To monitor long term warfarin therapy *after* stabilization (at least one week). NML: <2.0   Chronic atrial fibrillation 2.0-3.0
Tx DVT/PE   2.0-6.0
Heart valve replacement 2.5-3.5

Cardiac Profile

SGOT (AST)	7-21 U/L (♂)	SGOT *with MI* Onset 12-18 hours
	6-18 U/L (♀)	Peak 24-48 hours
		Duration 3-4 days
CK	38-174 U/L (♂)	CK *with MI* Onset 4-6 hours
	96-140 U/L (♀)	Peak 12-24 hours
		Duration 3-4 days
CK-MB	0 %	CK-MB *with MI* Onset 4-6 hours
		Peak 12-24 hours
		Duration 2-3 days
LDH	90-200 U/L	LDH *with MI* Onset 24-48 hours
		Peak 3-6 days
		Duration 7-10 days
LDH_1	17.5-28.3% total LDH	*With MI* $LDH_1 > LDH_2$
LDH_2	30.4-36.4% total LDH	Onset 12-24 hours
		Peak 48 hours
		Duration Variable
Troponin I Diagnostic level of MI 1.5ng/ml		**Positive** Suspect MI **Negative** Does not exclude diagnosis of unstable angina or MI of <7 hours duration

Urine Values

Specific Gravity	1.003-1.030	**PH**	4.5-8.0
Osmolality	300-1200 mOsm/L	**Volume** 1200 (600-2500cc/24hrs)	
Glucose	Normally not found	**Protein**	Normally not found
Bilirubin	Negative	**Urobilinogen** Up to 1.0 Ehrlich U	

HCG (pregnancy test) Negative: No HCG. Positive: HCG. HCG appears in the blood and urine 14 to 26 days after conception and peak in approximately 8 weeks. HCG is not found in non-pregnant women, in death of the fetus or after 3-4 days postpartum

❖ *Consistent appearance of* casts *and* epithelial cells *is abnormal*

While we are on the subject:

Urine Appearance	Clinical Condition
Pale, colorless	Diluted urine. Diabetes insipidus, alcohol ingestion, chronic kidney disease
Red, red brown	Hemoglobinuria, prophyrins, menstrual contamination. Drugs: Dilantin, Ex-Lax, thorazine, cascara, docusate Ca. Foods: Beets, rhubarb
Orange	Concentrated urine. ↓fluids, fever, ↑sweating. Drugs: Sulfonamides, Pyridium, Macrodantin. Foods: Rhubarb, carrots. Other: Carotene, bilirubin
Blue or green	Psudomonas toxemia. Drugs:Elavil, Robaxim, vitamin B complex, methylene blue, yeast concentrate
Brown or black	Lysol poisoning, melanin, bilirubin, methemoglobin, porphyrin. Drugs: Cascara, chloroquine, iron injectable compounds
Hazy, cloudy	Bacteria, pus, tissue, ↑WBCs, sperm, phosphates, uric acid
Milky	Pyuria, fat
Foam (large amount)	Severe cirrhosis of the liver

Cerebrospinal Fluid

Component	Result
Amount	(adults) 100-140ml
Appearance	Clear, colorless. Pink or red could be due to subarachnoid or cerebral hemorrhage or traumatic tap. Yellow might indicate old blood
Pressure	(on side) Newborn: 30-80 mmH$_2$O Children: 50-100mmH$_2$O Adults: 70-200mmH$_2$O. ↑pressure may be due to ↑ICP caused by meningitis, tumors or subarachnoid hemmorrhage
Cell count	Infants: 0-20/cu mm Adults: 0-10/cu mm
WBC	Differential: ↑neutrophils could be indicative of bacterial meningitis or cerebral abscess. ↑lymphocytes could be indicative of viral meningitis or encephalitis
Protein	Total:20-45 mg/dl Globulin:4-10mg/dl Albumin: 16-35mg/dl ↑protein levels may indicate infections/inflammation (meningitis, tumors or encephalitis)
Glucose	40-80mg/dl ↓levels may indicate bacterial meningitis, leukemia or tumors
Chloride	120-130 mEq/L (20 mEq/L higher than serum chloride)
Culture	Performed to determine type of organism present
Cytology	Performed to determine presence of cancerous cells

"The trouble with the rat race is that even if you win, you're still a rat."

Lily Tomlin

Drug Levels

Digoxin	1-2 ng/ml Toxic >2 ng/ml	**Phenytoin** (Dilantin)	10-20 µg/ml Toxic >20-30µg/ml Severe toxicity >40µg/ml
Theophylline	10-20 µg/ml	**Barbiturate coma** 10 mg/100ml	
Gentamicin	Trough 1-2 µg/ml Peak 6-8 µg/ml	**Tobramycin**	Trough 1-2 µg/ml Peak 6-8 µg/ml
Valporic Acid (Depakene)	50-100µg/ml Toxic >100µg/ml Severe toxicity >150µg/ml	**Warfarin** (Coumadin) 1-10µg/ml (adjusted usuallly by 1-2.5 x control) Toxic >10µg/ml	
Chlorpromazine (Thorazine)	50-300ng/ml Toxic >750ng/ml	**Haloperidol** (Haldol)	5-15ng/ml Toxic >50ng/ml
Morphine	10-80ng/ml Toxic >200ng/ml	**Methadone**	100-400ng/ml Toxic >2000ng/ml
Acetaminophen	Toxic >50µg/ml Hepatotoxicity >200µg/ml	**Lead**	Toxic >80µg/ml Urine >25µg/24
Ibuprofen	Toxic >100µg/ml	**Aspirin**	Toxic >500ng/ml
Diazepam (Valium)	0.5-2mg/L Toxic >3mg/L	**Lorazepam** (Ativan)	50-240ng/ml Toxic >300ng/ml
Lithium	0.8-1.2 mEq/L Toxic >1.5 mEq/L	**Amitriptyline** (Elavil)	110-225ng/ml Toxic >500ng/ml
Meperidine (Demerol)	0.4-0.7µg/ml Toxic >1.0µg/ml	**Verapamil**	100-300ng/ml Toxic >500ng/ml
Clonidine (Catapres)	0.2-2.0 ng/ml Toxic >2.0ng/ml	**Diltiazem** (Cardizem)	50-200ng/ml Toxic >200ng/ml

Units of Measurement

Temperature

$F - 32 \times 0.5555 = {}^{0}C$		${}^{0}C \times 1.8 + 32 = {}^{0}F$	
${}^{0}F$	${}^{0}C$	${}^{0}C$	${}^{0}F$
1	-17.7	1	32.0
106	35.0	41.0	95.0
107	35.5	35.6	95.9
108	36.1	42.0	96.8
109	36.6	36.6	97.5
110	37.2	43.0	98.6
111	37.7	37.6	99.5
112	38.3	44.0	100.4
113	38.8	38.6	101.3
114	39.4	45.0	102.2
115	40.0	39.6	103.1
116	40.5	46.0	104.0

Weight

$Lbs / 2.2 = Kgs$		$Kgs \times 2.2 = lbs$	
lb	Kg	Kg	lb
1	0.5	1	2.2
2	0.9	2	4.4
4	1.8	5	11
10	4.5	10	22
50	22.7	50	110
100	45.4	80	176
150	68.2	90	198
200	90.8	100	220

Equivalents of Measurement

Metric (volume)	Apothecary	Household
1 ml	15 minims	15 drops
15 ml	4 fluidrams	1 tablespoon
30 ml	1 fluid ounce	2 tablespoons
240 ml	8 fluid ounces	1 cup
480 ml (approx. 1/5 L)	1 pint	1 pint
960 ml (approx. 1 L)	1 quart	1 quart
3840 ml	1 gallon	1 gallon

French	Gauge	Millimeters	Centimeters	Inches
2.0	22	.667	.067	.026
2.5	21	.833	.083	.033
3.0	20	1.0	.10	.039
4.0	18	1.333	.133	.052
5.0	16	1.667	.167	.065
5.3	15	1.767	.177	.069
6.0	14	2.0	.20	.078
6.3	14	2.1	.21	.082
6.5	14	2.167	.217	.085
7.0	13	2.333	.233	.091
7.5	13	2.5	.25	.098
8.0	12	2.667	.267	.104
8.5	12	2.833	.283	.111
9.0	11	3.0	.30	.117
10.0	10	3.333	.333	.130
11.0	9	3.667	.367	.143
12.0	8	4.0	.40	.156
13.0	7	4.333	.433	.169
14.0	7	4.667	.467	.182

Notes:

Assessment

Quick E Critical Care Head-To-Toe Assessment

• Gather and review hx and meds form chart, kardex and report

• General appearance (loc, gait, mood, affect, speech, hearing), *how are you feeling, what is bothering you?* (open-ended questions)

• Head and neck (eye contact, pupils, skin condition, scalp, lips and tongue, cervical lymph nodes, neck vessels) *trouble swallowing, poor appetite, drinking O.K?*

• Upper extremities, inspect, patent pulses bilaterally, skin temp. and turgor, grasp, ROM, *any pain or trouble moving?*

• Anterior and posterior chest wall (inspect, palpate and auscultate). Listen for extra heart sounds, murmurs, thrills. Note heart rate and rhythm. Listen for adventitious breath sounds, *any chest pain or difficulty breathing?*

• Abdomen (first inspect, auscultate, then palpate). Note bowel sounds, presence of abdominal rigidity or enlarged organs. Light palpation first followed by deeper palpation. Rebound tenderness? ☛ Prominent aortic pulsation, or pulsation extending in the midline below umbilicus may indicate abdominal aneurysm. Do not attempt deep palpation in that area *Any pain, are bowels moving fine, are you voiding O.K.?*

• Lower extremities (patent pulses bilaterally, skin temp and turgor, capillary refill, assess strength by asking to push ball of foot against your hand, ROM, note any edema, obvious deformities? *any problems moving, any calf tenderness, numbness?*

Italics are questions for conscious client. Refer to other portions of the book for specific techniques.

Abdominopelvic Quadrants

RUQ
Liver
Gallbladder
Pylorus
Head of pancreas
Duodenum
Upper right kidney

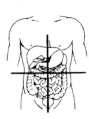

LUQ
Left lobe of liver
Spleen
Stomach
Body of pancreas
Left kidney

RLQ
Lower right kidney
Cecum
Appendix
Ascending colon
R fallopian tube (E)
R ovary (E)
R ureter, Bladder (distended)

LLQ
Descending colon
Sigmoid colon
L ureter
Bladder (distended)
L fallopian tube (E)
L ovary (E)

Assessment Scales

Pitting Edema		Pulse	
+1	5mm depth	0	Absent
+2	8-10 mm depth	+1	Decreased, thready
+3	> 10 mm depth, up to 30 sec	+2	Normal
+4	>20 mm depth, longer than 30 sec	+3	Full, bounding
Deep Tendon Reflexes		**Muscle Movement of Extremities**	
0	Absent	0	No contraction
1+	Diminished	1	Slight contraction
2+	Normal	2	Active with gravity eliminated
3+	Increased	3	Active with gravity
4+	Hyperactive, clonus	4	Active, some resistance
		5	Full strength against resistance

Rule of Nines

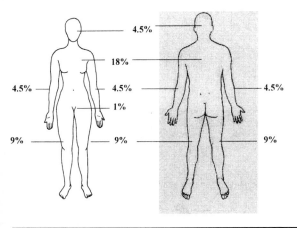

Infants and small children: Head, anterior trunk and posterior trunk each 18%. Arms each 9%. Legs each 14%
Children: Head 14%. Anterior trunk and posterior trunk each 18%. Arms each 9%. Legs each 16%.

Diabetic Ketoacidosis vs. Hyperglycemic Hyperosmolar Nonketotic Coma

Characteristics	DKA	HHNC
Cause	Insufficient exogenous insulin for glucose needs, as in non-compliance to type I DM, or ↑demand from illness, surgery or activity. Sudden onset (hours to days)	Insufficient exogenous/endogenous insulin for glucose needs. Insulin resistance and insulin deficiency produce hyperglycemia. Usually affected: type II DM >65 y/o. Insidious onset (days to weeks)
S & S	Lethargy, Kussmaul respirations, fruity odor. N+V, abdominal pain, orthostasis, cerebral edema. Many patients are hypotensive, tachycardic with mild to moderate volume depletion	Profound dehydration. Patient usually stuporous. May manifest neuro deficits (cranial nerve abnormalities, abnl reflexes, seizures). Usually hypotensive with nml to diminished resp. Cerebral edema is rare
Serum glucose	300-800mg/dl	600-2000mg/dl
Serum ketones	Strongly positive	Normal to mild ↑
Serum osmolality	<350mOsm/l	>350mOsm/l
Urine acetone	Strong	Absent or mild
Mortality	8-10%	12-50%

Cardiac

Cardiac Assessment

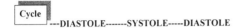

Cycle ---DIASTOLE------SYSTOLE-----DIASTOLE

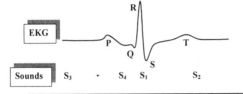

EKG

Sounds S_3 · S_4 S_1 S_2

Murmur Scale

Grade	Description
I	Barely audible
II	Audible
III	Moderately loud, no thrill
IV	Loud, no thrill
V	Very loud, associated with a thrill
VI	Very loud, thrill, audible with Stethoscope off the chest

Heart Sounds

S_1	Beginning systole. Loudest at apex. Caused by closure of AV valves
S_2	Loudest at base. Caused by closure of semilunar valves
S_3	May be normal when in children and young adults. Associated with CHF. Abnormal over age 35 termed *ventricular gallop*
S_4	May occur in adults >40 without disease. Pathologic S_4 termed *atrial gallop*

Assessing the Cardiovascular System: Palpation

Upper Extremities Brachial and radial pulses, temperature, capillary refill
Neck Carotid pulses (listen for bruits first)
Precordium Apical pulse, other chest pulsations (thrills, heaves)
Abdomen Femoral pulses, abdominal aortic pulse
Lower Extremities Popliteal, posterior tibial and dorsalis pedis pulses. Edema or phlebitis present?

Pacemaker Terminology

Fixed-rate *(asynchronous)* Paces at fixed rate regardless of spontaneous cardiac activity

Demand *(synchronous)* Paces only when heart's intrinsic pacemaker fails to function at a predetermined rate.

AV Sequential *(dual-chamber pacing)* Paces both atrium and ventricle in sequence

Pacemaker Codes

Code	Description	Code	Description
AOO	Atrial (A) fixed rate, no sensing	AAT	A demand, paced/sensed, triggered response to sensing
VOO	Ventricular (V) fixed rate, no sensing	VAT	AV synchronous, V pacing, A sensing, triggered response
DOO	AV sequential fixed, no sensing	DVI	AV sequential, A+V pacing, V sensing, inhibited response
VVI	V demand, V paced/sensed, inhibited response to sensing	VDD	A synchronous, V inhibited, V pacing, A+V sensing, inhibited response to sensing in V and triggered response to sensing in A
VVT	V demand, V paced/sensed, triggered response to sensing		
AAI	A demand, paced/sensed, inhibited response to sensing	DDD	Universal, A+V senses and paced inhibited in V, triggered in A

"The only tyrant I accept in this world is the still voice within."

Mahatma Gandhi

Quick-E Electrocardiogram Guide

• An EKG (ECG) records electrical impulses of the heart which normally originate at the sinoatrial (SA) node traveling across the R atrium and to the atrioventricular (AV) node (depolarization of the atria, "**P**" wave). The impulse travels down the septum (bundle of His and bundle branches) to the Purkinje fibers (depolarizing the ventricles, "**QRS** complex").
Repolarization of the ventricles accounts for the "**T**" wave.

• EKG leads are used to "capture" this electrical activity. Each lead has 3 electrodes (positive, negative and ground). If wave of depolarization travels toward positive electrode, a positive deflection is recorded on the EKG paper (above isoelectric line). If wave of depolarization travels away from positive electrode, a negative deflection is recorded on the EKG paper (below isoelectric line). When depolarization travels perpendicular to positive electrode, a biphasic complex occurs. Different leads, therefore, take different "pictures" of the electrical activity in the heart.

• The EKG paper records both the speed and magnitude of cardiac electrical impulses. When measured horizontally, each small box is equivalent to 0.04 seconds; each large box 0.2 seconds. When measured vertically, each small box is 0.1 mV and each large box 0.5 mV (measurements of strength of force).

• The electrical impulse, as it travels through the ventricles, tends to go in a certain direction. The fancy name is the *mean vector*. When the mean vector is plotted in a graph, it is called the *hexaxial reference system* and a degree can be assigned to it for more precise measurement. This degree represents the *ventricular axis*. Normal range for the ventricular axis is about −30 to +110. When a MI occurs and tissue dies, or when electrical activity originates in other than "normal" places (*ectopic beats*), the direction of electrical impulses going through the heart will obviously be affected. Thus, *axis deviation* is used as a criterion to help diagnose cardiac problems.

The Normal EKG

Component	Criteria
Rate	Atrial = Ventricular. 60-100/min.
Rhythm	Regular. R-R and P-P vary < 0.16sec.
P wave	Present, one per QRS
PR interval	0.12-0.20 sec. and constant
QRS	0.06-0.10 sec. >0.12, bundle branch block
ST segment	Flat (isoelectric). Should not be depressed > 0.05mm. May be elevated <1mm in limb leads and <2mm in some precordial leads. ↑ST suggests vasospasm or acute injury. ↓ST suggests ischemia
QT interval	0.30-0.40 sec. Prolonged interval associated with torsade de pointes
T wave	<10mm in precordial leads, <5mm in limb leads. Tall T associated with hyperkalemia, ischemia
U wave	<0.24 sec., 2.5mm max. ↑in hypokalemia

Calculating Rate

Count number of R waves in a 6 sec. Strip x 10 (preferred method if irregular rhythm)
Count number of large boxes between 2 R waves and divide by 300
Count number of small boxes between 2 R waves and divide by 1500

Axis in Lead II

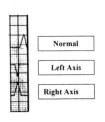

Normal

Left Axis

Right Axis

Causes of L Axis Deviation: Normal variation, Mechanical shifts (high diaphragm), L anterior hemiblock, L vent. hypertrophy. Wolff-Parkinson-White syndrome, cardiomyopathy, hyperkalemia.

Causes of R Axis Deviation: Normal variation, mechanical shifts, L posterior hemiblock, R vent. hypertrophy, lateral wall MI, RBBB, dextrocardia

Location of Infarction and EKG Patterns

Location	Leads Involved	EKG Pattern
Inferior wall	II, III, aV$_F$	Abnormal Q, ST↑, T inversion
Anterior wall	I, aV$_L$,V$_{2-4}$	Abnormal Q, loss of R progression, ST↑, T inversion
Posterior wall	Mirror image changes in V$_{1-3}$	Tall R, ST depression, tall symmetrical T
Lateral wall	V$_{4-6}$, I, aV$_L$	Abnormal Q, ST↑, T inversion
Right ventricle	V$_4$R, V$_5$R ,V$_6$R	ST elevation >1mm

Differentiating Wide QRS

No P waves?	All negative in V$_6$ = V tach Bizarre axis = V tach
PR < .12 sec?	Wolff-Parkinson-White syndrome
Total QRS prolonged?	Quinidine or procainamide toxicity, severe hyperkalemia
Initial QRS peaked in V$_1$-V$_6$?	RBBB
QRS wide overall in V$_1$-V$_6$?	LBBB
LBBB with axis < -45 degrees?	Left anterior hemiblock (LAHB)
LBBB with axis > 120 degrees?	Left posterior hemiblock (LPHB)

Differentiating Prolonged PR Intervals

P with every QRS?	1st degree heart block
Progressive PR prolongation?	2nd degree heart block (type I, Wenckebach)
Constant PR with dropped beats?	2nd degree heart block (type II)
No relationship between P waves and QRS?	3rd degree heart block

Assessment of Jugular Vein Distention

• JVD occurs with ↑central venous pressure and it is characteristic of R sided heart failure. To assess for JVD:

   • Have client reclined at 30-45 degree angle
   • To visualize vein, turn clients head slightly to the L. If jugular vein is not visible, apply light finger pressure across the sternocleidomastoid muscle (above and parallel to clavicle). The obstruction of flow will fill the external jugular vein. Once location has been identified, release pressure and continue with assessment
   • Ask client to exhale and measure
   • Measure from horizontal imaginary baseline extending from the sternum (sternal angle). See figure next page
   • Fullness in the vein extending >3cm above sternal angle is evidence of ↑venous pressure
   • Document findings to include the HOB angle

• Estimating central venous pressure:

   • Observe for the highest point of pulsation along internal jugular vein (this vein runs anterior and parallel to external jugular vein) during exhalation
   • Vertical distance between pulsation and the sternal angle is estimated
   • Add 5 to that number and that is your estimated central venous pressure in cm's (NML: 3-8cm water or 2-4mmHg)
   • Document findings to include the HOB angle

Note: Some authorities feel that estimation of central venous pressure as above is often inaccurate and thus not good in predicting elevated pressures. They propose that the only accurate statement is that right atrial pressure is high when there is neck vein distention up to the jaw margin while the client is seated at 90 degrees. Right atrial pressure is generally >15mmHg at this point.

Assessment of Jugular Vein Distention (cont.)

● **Hepatojugular Reflux** (also known as abdominal compression) Clients with R ventricular failure have livers with dilated sinusoids. Pressure on liver pushes blood from these sinusoids causing further neck vein distention. To perform, client has to be lying in bed, breathing normal and with mouth open to prevent a Valsalva maneuver. Place firm, progressive pressure over liver (RUQ) with hand for 10 seconds. **NML:** Internal and external jugular veins show transient distention early, followed by a return to baseline during later part of compression. **ABNL:** Veins remain distended during the entire period of compression and fall rapidly upon sudden release of compression (R ventricular failure, ↑pulmonary artery wedge pressure)

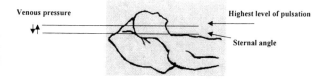

"Say what you want about long dresses, but they cover a multitude of shins."

Mae West

Notes:

Cranial Nerves

Cranial Nerve	Type	Function	Assessment
I Olfactory	Sensory	Smell	Test with non-noxious smells such as orange, coffee, soap or vanilla
II Optic	Sensory	Vision	Visual acuity
III Oculomotor	Mixed	Ocular movement, pupil constriction, lens shape, eyelids	Check pupils for size, light reaction and accommodation. Assess extraocular movements
IV Trochlear	Motor	Eye movement	
V Trigeminal	Mixed	Chewing, sensation of face, cornea, scalp, mouth and nose	Palpate chewing muscles as client clenches teeth. Check for sensation on face
VI Abducens	Motor	Lateral eye movement	*
VII Facial	Mixed	Taste on anterior tongue, facial muscles, close eye, saliva, tears	Lift eyebrows, smile. Identify taste of safe substance (lemon, salt)
VIII Acoustic	Sensory	Hearing and balance	Hearing acuity
IX Glossopharyngeal	Mixed	Gag reflex, taste on posterior tongue, swallowing, parotid gland, carotid reflex	Assess uvula and soft palate placement with tongue depress while client says "ahh." Uvula to midline. Note gag reflex.
X Vagus	Mixed	Talking and swallowing, general carotid sensation, sinus, and reflex	
XI Spinal	Motor	Trapezius and sternomastoid movement	Shrug shoulders. Rotate head to sides against resistance.
XII Hypoglossal	Motor	Tongue movement	Note speech. Midline forward thrust of tongue

* Assessed together with cranial nerves III and IV

Neurologic Reference

Sign	Description
Babinski	Sole of foot is stroked. Abnormal: Dorsiflexion of big toe and fanning of the toes Upper motor neuron dysfunction. Normal: Plantar flexion
Brudzinski	Passive neck flexion trigger flexion of the hip and knee. Pathologic reflex indicating meningeal irritation
Kernig	Resistance to full extension of the leg at the knee when the hip is flexed. Pathologic reflex indicating meningeal irritation
Oculocephalic (doll's eye maneuver)	Head rotated from side to side. Abnormal: Eyes move with the head fixed in place. This is a normal response in newborns but disappears as ocular fixation develops. Indicates brainstem injury. Normal: Eyes remain in the initial position, then turn slowly in the direction of head rotation
Oculovestibular (ice water calorics, also called Barany's test)	Ear alternately irrigated with hot and cold water. Abnormal: *Supratentorial or metabolic lesion*, eyes move slowly toward irrigated ear and remain there for 2-3 minutes. Absent fast return to midline. *Brainstem lesion*, downward deviation and rotary jerking of one eye. *Severe brainstem injury*, no response. Normal: Hot water irrigation produces a rotatory nystagmus towards irrigated ear. Cold water produces a rotatory nystagmus away from irrigated ear
Decorticate	Flexion of upper extremities, legs may be extended. Indicates lesion to the mesencephalic region of the brain
Decerebrate	Extension of upper extremities with internal rotation, legs may be extended. Indicates brainstem lesion

- **Spinal Cord** 31 Pairs of spinal nerves originate from the cord: 8 cervical, 12 thoracic, 5 lumbar, 5 sacral, 1 coccygeal. Lesions below first thoracic vertebra may produce *paraplegia*. Lesions above first thoracic vertebra may produce *quadriplegia*. Lesions that completely transect the spinal cord cause loss of motor and sensory function below the level of injury.

- **Dysreflexia** state in which an individual with a sc injury at T7 or above experiences a life threatening uninhibited sympathetic response of the nervous system to a noxious stimulus. S+S include pallor below the injury, red splotches on skin above the injury, paroxysmal hypertension (sudden periodic ↑BP systolic >140 and diastolic >90mm Hg), headache, blurred vision, chest pain, horner's syndrome, metallic taste in mouth, gooseflesh formation when skin is cooled. Treatment: Elevate head, identify and remove noxious stimulus (bladder or bowel distention, skin irritation etc), monitor BP closely, have available antihypertensives as physician prescribes.

Glasgow Coma Scale

Eyes Open:	Score
Spontaneously	4
To Verbal Command	3
To Pain	2
No Response	1
Best Motor Response To Verbal Command:	
Obeys	6
To Painful Stimulus:	
Localizes Pain	5
Flexion-Withdrawal	4
Flexion-Abnormal	3
Extension	2
No Response	1
Best Verbal Response	
Oriented and converses	5
Disoriented and converses	4
Inappropriate Words	3
Incomprehensible Sounds	2
No Response	1
GCS Total	3-15

Pupil Gauge (mm)

2 3 4   5   6   7   8   9

• • •   ●   ●   ●   ⬤   ⬤

Notes:

Respiratory

Oxygen Delivery Systems

Nasal Cannula	4-6 L/min deliver 35-40% FIo_2. Higher flow rates dry airway mucosa and not recommended
Simple Mask	Minimum flow of 5-6 L/min. 10-12 L/min deliver 55-65% Fio_2
Nonrebreathing Mask	Attached reservoir allows theoretical delivery of 90-100% FIo_2. In practice, usually delivers up to 70% FIo_2 at 10 L/min
Venturi Mask	Delivers controlled Fio_2 at specific rates. 4 L/min (24%), 6 L/min (28%), 8 L/min (35%) and 10 L/min (40% FIo_2)

Adventitious Sounds

Crackles	Air that contains serous secretions. Bubbling, wet sound (a.k.a. rales). Pneumonia, CHF, bronchitis, emphysema
Wheezes	Air flowing through narrow airways. High pitch, muscial quality. Acute asthma, bronchitis
Stridor	High pitch, crowing sound. Croup, airway obstruction, acute epiglotitis (children)
Rub	Coarse and low pitch. Pleuritis

Assess

Pitch	Is it high or low?
Timing	When is it occurring? Late or early? Inspiratory or expiratory?
Quality	Is it loud or soft? Coarse or fine? Is it continuous or intermittent?
Location	Where on the chest wall was sound auscultated?

"Anybody who has an identity problem had better wise up and get with the program!"

Jack Handey

Chest Tube Placement and Indications

Indications for Chest Tubes	Position
•Mechanically ventilated clients with any size pneumothorax or hemothorax •Open/Closed pneumothorax >20% •Hemothorax >500ml •Pnemohemothorax •Pleural effusion	•To drain fluid: posteriorly, midaxillary line at the 4th or 5th intercostal space •To release air: anteriorly midclavicular line at second intercostal space

Chest Tube Drainage

Water Seal Chamber	Collection Chamber	Suction Chamber
Usual level at 2-3 cm. Bubbling indicates air leak in system. If bubbling, clamp near client. If bubbling stops, leak within client or at insertion site. Notify physician. If bubbling does not stop, leak is in the system. Locate leak by clamping along tubing. Replace and retape equipment prn	If drainage >100 ml/hr for 2 hours or sudden change in amount of bloody drainage, notify physician. If drainage is decreased, check for kinks and clots. Consult your local protocol in regards to milking tube	Usual 15-25 cm water. Maintain constant, gentle bubbling. Maintain appropriate fluid level. ☞ Keep a bottle of sterile water and sterile petroleum gauze available. If system interrupted, tube should be placed in a few cms of sterile water while system reestablished. Gauze for applying to chest wall if tube is accidentally removed

☞*6 hours of bleeding at 200ml/hr or 12 hours at 100ml/hr is indication for operative intervention*

ABG's

pH	7.35-7.45	Pao$_2$	80-100 mm Hg*
Paco$_2$	35-45 mm Hg	HCO$_3$	22-26 mEq/L
% Sat	95-99	Base Excess	+/-2

*If client >60 years old, Pao$_2$ = 80 mm Hg – 1 mm Hg for every year over 60

Interpreting ABGs		
PH	If ↑ Alkalosis	If ↓ Acidosis
Paco$_2$	If ↑Hypoventilation, respiratory acidosis or compensating metabolic alkalosis	If ↓ Hyperventilation, respiratory alkalosis or compensating for metabolic acidosis
HCO$_3$	If ↑ Metabolic alkalosis or compensating for respiratory acidosis	If ↓ Metabolic acidosis or compensating for respiratory alkalosis

Type of Imbalance		
Respiratory Disorder	If pH↑ and Paco$_2$↓	or	If pH↓ and Paco$_2$↑
Metabolic Disorder	If pH↑ and HCO$_3$↑	or	If pH↓ and HCO$_3$↓
Compensating	If Paco$_2$↑ and HCO$_3$↑	or	If Paco$_2$↓ and HCO$_3$↓
Mixed Disorder	If Paco$_2$↑ and HCO$_3$↓	or	If Paco$_2$↓ and HCO$_3$↑

"Whoever gossips to you will gossip about you."

Spanish Proverb

Intubation Guidelines

Tube Size (adult)		Cuff Pressure
Orotracheal	Nasotracheal	>20mmHg ↑risk for tracheal damage
♂ 8-8.5mm i.d.	<7.5mm i.d.	<15mmHg ↑risk for aspiration
♀ 7-8mm i.d.		

Intubation Attempt
Position with neck flexed and head slightly extended (sniff)
Suction oropharynx and remove any dental devices
Preoxygenate with 100% O_2
Attempt limited to 30 seconds

After Insertion
Assess for bilateral chest sounds and bilateral chest movement
Auscultate epigastric area (gurgling sounds indicate esophageal intubation.
Remove tube and reintubate)
Cuffing: Minimal occlusive technique
Place stethoscope over larynx and slowly remove air in amounts of 0.2ml
until air leak is heard. Slowly reinsert air until inspiratory leak stops
Secure tube and obtain chest x-ray to confirm placement

After Securing Tube
After final adjustment of position, note level of insertion
Check tube periodically for displacement
Avoid excessive negative pressure when suctioning (-80 to −120mmHg)
Avoid unnecessary suction and tube manipulation
Support and stabilize tube when moving/suctioning
Avoid frequent retaping
Sedate prn to minimize risk of self-extubation

"Always bear in mind that your own resolution to succeed is more important than any one thing."

Abraham Lincoln

Extubation Guidelines

- Suction airway, mouth and pharynx
- Undo ties/tape securing tube and fully deflate cuff
- Hyperoxygenate before removing (give several breaths via bag)
- Swiftly remove tube
- After removal of tracheostomy tube, cover stoma with a dry, sterile dressing. Stoma should close within several days

Mechanical Ventilation

- **Inidications include:**
  - Respiratory Rate > 35
  - Maximal inspiratory pressure < 20mmHg
  - Vital capacity < 10ml/kg
  - Minute ventilation < 3 or > 20L/min
  - $Paco_2$ > 50mmHg with pH < 7.25
  - Pao_2 < 55mmHg (with supplementary O_2)
  - Alveolar-arterial Oxygen tension difference (with 100% O_2) > 450mmHg
  - Negative inspiratory force < -25cmH$_2$O
- Look for other clinical signs including alterations in vital signs (↑ or ↓ pulse, BP, RR), cyanosis, dysrhythmias, nasal flaring, altered respiratory patterns and intercostal retractions

"Death is more universal than life; everyone dies but not everyone lives."

A. Sachs

Vent Settings (adult)

Respiratory Rate: Delivered breaths per minute	
Tidal Volume: Volume delivered during breath (usually 10-15ml/kg)	
O_2 Concentration: (Fio_2) between 21-100%	
I:E Ratio: Inspiratory to expiratory time ratio. Adjusted with inspiratory flow rate (usually 1:2 unless inverse ratio ventilation is in use)	
Inspiratory Flow Rate: Peak Flow. Flow of tidal volume delivery	
Sensitivity: Adjusts vent response to patient's respiratory effort in certain vent modes. Sets amount of effort patient must generate to initiate breath	
Sigh: A big breath used to simulate normal sigh to prevent alveoli collapse (usually 1.5-2 times tidal volume with rate of 4-5 times per hour)	
Pressure Limits: Sets maximal pressure vent will generate. If limit is reached, ventilator will spill undelivered volume outside patient –and sound alarm. Limit usually set at 10-20cmH$_2$O above normal peak pressure. Low pressure setting will alarm when specified pressure parameters are not reached (see trouble-shooting)	

Vent Modes*

CMV Controlled Mode Ventilation	Delivers volume and rate at preset setting regardless of patient's effort. Used primarily on apneic patients. Spontaneously breathing patients must be sedated and/or paralyzed
A/C Assist Control	Breath delivered at preset volume in response to patient's inspiratory effort. Will initiate breath if patient apneic. Primarily used in spontaneously breathing patients with weak respiratory muscles
SIMV Synchronous Intermittent Mandatory Ventilation	Vent breaths are synchronized with patient's respiratory effort. May ↑ breathing work and promote fatigue
PEEP Positive End Expiratory Pressure	Positive expiratory pressure applied during vent breaths. Useful in patients with acute diffuse restrictive lung disease and hypoxemic refractory to oxygen therapy. Used with CMV, A/C, or SIMV

CPAP Constant Positive Airway Pressure	Similar to PEEP except that it maintains positive airway pressure throughout respiratory cycle not just expiration. Used as a primary mode of ventilation. Useful for weaning *NG helps Ē GI Bleed lessens pressure to gut*
PSV Positive Support Ventilation	Patient controls rate, inspiratory flow and tidal volume. Provides positive pressure only in response to spontaneous breath. Can be used with SIMV to support spontaneous breaths and as a weaning tool to ↓ breathing work and fatigue
HFV High Frequency Ventilation	Different types with different delivery rates. Vents deliver small volume of gas at rapid rates. Used in situations in which conventional mechanical ventilation compromises hemodynamic stability, with diseases that create a risk of barotrauma, and with brohchopleural fistulas
IRV Inverse- Ratio Ventilation	Ventilation in which proportion of inspiratory time to expiratory time is ≥ 1:1 (longer inspiration than expiration). Used in patients with hypoxemia refractory to PEEP
NNPPV Nocturnal Nasal Positive Pressure Ventilation	Positive pressure delivered via nasal mask. Used at night for patients with respiratory muscle weakness or nighttime hypoventilation

* Different brands of ventilators will have different features. Not all modes are available on all ventilators. Consult user manual

Vent Weaning Criteria

Fio_2	< 50%
Vital Capacity	> 10-15ml/kg
Tidal Volume	> 5ml/kg
Respiratory Rate	12-20 breaths/min.
PEEP	< 5cmH$_2$O
Minute Ventilation	< 10L/min
Negative Inspiratory Force	> -25cmH$_2$O
$PaCO_2$	Within patients normal range
PaO_2	> 60mmHg on Fio$_2$ of < 50%

Troubleshooting the Vent

Alarm	Implications
High pressure	√ Patient for secretions and, or biting ET tube. √ ET tube or trache placement. √ tubing for kinks and water accumulation. Reposition patient if needed. Assess breath sounds (rule out bronchospasm, pneumothorax etc.)
Low volume or pressure	Ensure patient is connected to vent. Assess patient's breathing effort (initiated breaths, breath sounds), √ for loose connections. √ for cuff leaks.

Terminology

Afterload: Resistance against which L ventricle must eject its volume of blood during contraction. About 90% of Oxygen required by myocardium is consumed in the afterload effort

Allen Test: To assess collateral circulation before radial artery cannulation. Client makes a fist while nurse compresses ulnar and radial arteries until hand blanches. Client opens hand, release one of the arteries and hand should immediately turn pink. Repeat on other artery

Cardiac Output: Volume of blood ejected from the heart over 1 min. Cardiac output, expressed in liters/min. = heart rate (HR) in beats/min. multiplied by stroke volume (SV) in milliliters per beat. CO=HR x SV Determinants of CO include preload, afterload, contractility and HR

Contractility: (inotropy) Force of the heart contraction when preload and afterload are constant (see Sterling's Law of the Heart)

Dicrotic Notch: May be present on down stroke of arterial wave form and represents closure of the aortic valves and the beginning of diastole

Ejection Fraction: Ratio of the stroke volume from the left ventricle per beat to the volume of blood in the left ventricle at the end of diastole (LVEDV). Used as clinical index to measure cardiac contractility and function. NML >50%. <30% indicative of poor ventricular function, poor ventricular filling or obstruction to outflow, or a combination of these

"A doctor can bury his mistakes but an architect can only advise his client to plant vines."

Frank Lloyd Wright

Phlebostatic Axis: Reference point along the chest used as a baseline for consistent transducer height placement. To obtain axis, draw an imaginary line from the fourth intercostal space at the right side of the sternum to an intersection with the midaxillary line. This is the approximate level of the R atrium and the location for transducer placement

Pulsus Alternans: (alternating pulse) Regular alteration of weak and strong pulsations. Sometimes seen in patients with advanced L ventricular failure

Pulsus Paradoxus: (paradoxical pulse) ↓>10mmHg in arterial waveform that occurs during inhalation. May be a sign of pericardial tamponade, constrictive pericarditis, severe lung disease, or advanced heart failure

Starling's Law of the Heart: Force of the heartbeat is determined by length of fibers comprising the myocardial walls. Contractility↑ as result of ↑volume until a maximal point. After reaching this point, excessive stretching causes contractility to ↓

Stroke Volume: Amount of blood ejected from the ventricles during a ventricular contraction

Thermodilution: A method for testing CO. Small amounts of a cold liquid (normal saline) is injected into the proximal lumen of a PA catheter (Swan-Ganz). The temperature change is recorded by a thermister at a point farther along the bloodstream. CO is calculated as a function of the flow rate of the saline solution multiplied by a factor derived from the temperature differences

Transducer: Receives the physiologic signal from the catheter and converts it into electrical energy suitable for transmission over monitoring devices. Must be placed at phlebostatic axis for accurate reading. If placed below phlebostatic axis, false-high reading obtained and if placed above, false-low reading obtained.

Flow Directed Pulmonary Artery Catheter
Waveforms and Pressures

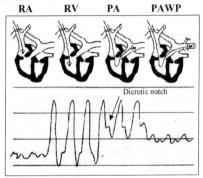

RA Nml (mmHg)	RV Nml (mmHg)	PA Nml (mmHg)	PAWP Nml: (mmHg)
Mean 0-8	Systolic: 15-28 Diastolic: 0-8	Systolic: 15-30 Diastolic: 5-15 Mean: 10-20	4-12
If ↑ : ?RV failure, tricuspid stenosis/re-gurgitation, pulmonary htn, LV failure	If ↑ : ?mitral stenosis, CHF, LV failure, pulmonary disease, AV septal defect	If ↑: ?LV failure, ↑pulmo. Bloodflow, ↑pulmo. Arteriolar resistance	If ↑:?LV failure, mitral stenosis/ insuffi-ciency

❖ Low pressures associated with hypovolemic states. See *Cardiac Formulas* for calculations and parameters of more hemodynamic values

Troubleshooting Arterial and PA Lines

Problem	Troubleshooting
Air bubbles	√ connections, tighten if needed, √for damaged stopcocks, √ flush
Blood in tubing	Flush system out, ensure connections are tight and stopcocks in correct position
Can not flush line	√ for kinks, ensure stopcocks in correct position, √ pressure on flush solution (about 300mmHg). If clot is suspected, aspirate gently with small syringe at proximal stopcock and flush once clot is removed
Damping of waveform	√ for kinks, air or blood in system. √ pressure on flush solution (about 300mmHg) and ensure heparin solution concentration and rate are correct. Attempt to aspirate and flush line with fast flush valve device. With PA line have patient cough
False low	√ transducer placement. √ for air in system and ensure all connections tight. Recalibrate
False high	√ transducer placement. √ for air in system. √ heparin flush rate. Recalibrate
Hemorrhage	√ for loose connection or open stopcock. Once blood leak eliminated, tighten all connections, flush line and estimate blood loss
No waveform	√ power, √ gain, √ transducer placement, √ stopcocks and all connections and cables. √ for blood/air in system. Consider changing transducer

Troubleshooting Arterial and PA Lines (PA Lines Only)

Problem	Troubleshooting
Continuous RV waveform	√ with previous tracings. Reposition patient. Attempt to float catheter into PA by inflating balloon. If unsuccessful, catheter will need to be repositioned or pulled back into RA*
Continuous PAWP waveform	√ with previous tracings. √ inflation port (ballon should be deflated). Reposition patient. If unsuccessful, catheter will need to be pulled back*
↑ ventricular ectopy	√ tracing to rule out RV placement. See above. Administer antidysrhythmics as ordered

*Note: Please check facility guidelines for protocols and procedures

❖ If ever in doubt about accuracy of arterial waveform, *take a cuff blood pressure* and attempt to correlate

"Nobody grows old merely by living a number of years. We grow old by deserting our ideals. Years may wrinkle the skin, but to give up enthusiasm wrinkles the soul."

Samuel Ullman

Intraaortic Balloon Pump Device (IABP)*

Description: Temporary mechanical circulation assist device used to support the failing heart through diastolic augmentation and afterload reduction. Usually inserted into descending thoracic aorta or the femoral artery (percutaneously). After proper synchronization with patient's EKG pattern, device functions by inflating during diastole and deflating just before systole

Indications: Left ventricular failure. Unstable angina when angina and dysrhythmias persistent and refractory to drugs, especially when coronary angiography or possible revascularization can not be performed in timely and/or safe manner

Complications: Aortic dissection, femoral artery laceration, hematomas, femoral neuropathies, renal failure from renal artery occlusion, arterial thrombi and emboli, limb ischemia and line sepsis

General Considerations: Monitor EKG/balloon timing. Monitor for dysrhythmias. MAP should be maintained at about 80mmHg with adequate pumping. Monitor peripheral pulses and adequate perfusion distal to insertion. Monitor/assess L radial pulse and urine output carefully (rule out migration of catheter and arterial occlusion). Patient at complete bed rest with HOB↑ at 30 degrees max. Prevent flexion of involved hip. Log-roll reposition q2hr. Monitor bleeding, platelet count. Strict sterile dressing changes. Administer cardiac drugs, anticoagulants and prophylactic antibiotics as Rx

* This quick guide is aimed as a general familiarization with the subject. Management of the client with an IABP, and of the pumping console and equipment should be performed by specially trained personnel.

IABP Counterpulsation Timing

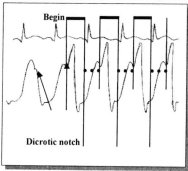

Inflate
(at dicrotic notch)
Deflate
(at end diastole)
Inflation/deflation triggered
by R wave in EKG tracing.
Inflation ↑aortic pressure
↑myocardial O_2 supply and
↑systemic perfusion. Deflation
↓ myocardial O_2 demands by
↓ afterload allowing L
ventricle
to eject at lower pressures

IABP Weaning Criteria

- **Hemodynamic stability with no or minimal drug support**
- **CI ≥ 2L/min/m²**
- **Systolic BP ≥ 100mmHg**
- **Absence of crackles, S₃**
- **PAWP** <18-20mmHg
- **U/O ≥ 30ml/hr**
- **HR** <110bpm

Dependence on balloon >48 hours usually indicative of severe cardiac dysfunction and associated with poor prognosis

Notes:

Dosage Formulas

* *Amount to administer*

  (Dose ordered / Dose on hand) x Amount on hand =Amount to administer

  e.g. Order: 100mg Theophylline po q6h. Have 200mg per tablet.
  $(100/200) = 0.5$ X 1 tablet = 0.5 (1/2 tablet)

* *Hourly Rate*

  Total volume / Total # of hours infusing = Hourly rate

  e.g. Order: Infuse 1000ml NaCl over 12 hours
  $1000/12 = 83.3$ ml/hr (pump rate)

* Determine drops per minute

  (Total volume x Drop factor) / Time in minutes = Drops per minute

  <u>Drop Factor</u>: Microdrip Infusion Set: 60gtt/min.

                    Macrodrip Infusion Set: 15gtt/min.

  If in doubt, look at the infusion set package, it will tell you the drop factor

  e.g. Order: Infuse 1000ml NaCl over 12 hours

  $(83.3X60)/60 = 83$gtt/min

  or same order with a macrodrip

  $(83.3X 15)/60 = 21$gtt/min

* Determine Concentration

  e.g. Order: Patient's IV fluids has 25,000 units of Heparin in 500cc of ½ NS.

  25,000u/500cc = 50 units/cc

* To determine rate for dose per hour

  e.g. Order: Administer 90 mg of Theophylline per hour. The IV fluids hanging are 1000mg of Theophylline in 250cc of D5 ½ NS.

  Concentration = 1000mg/250cc = 4mg/cc

  Dose per hour = 90 mg per hour/4mg per cc = 22.5 cc (rate for pump)

Dosage Formulas (cont.)

* *Determining mcg/Kg/minute* (don't panic! Work it step by step)
  Determine Rate/Determine Dose

  > *Example: Dopamine 400 mg in 250cc D5W. Pt weighs 200 lbs.*
  > *Order: Start Dopamine at 10 mcg/Kg/min.*

  b. *Determining rate:*
  1. Covert lbs to <u>kg</u> (in our example, pt weighs 91Kg)
  2. Determine <u>concentration</u> of solution (400 mg Dopamine in 250cc D5w is 400mg/250cc = 1.6mg/cc)
  3. Convert mg to <u>mcg</u> (1mg=1000mcg, 1.6mg = 1600mcg)
  4. **Rate (cc/hr): (mcg X Kg X 60) / concentration (mcg/cc)**
  (in our example: (10mcg X 91 Kg X 60) / 1600mcg/cc = 34cc per hour)

  b. Determining Dose:
      What if, using our example above, the rate was decreased from 34cc/hr to 25cc/hr. What would the dosage be? (How many mcg/kg/min of dopamine is our fellow above now getting?)
  1. **Dose = (New rate)X(Concentration in mcg/cc) / (KgX60)**
  (in our example: 25(cc/hr our new rate)X(1600mcg/cc) / 91KgX60min
           = 7.3 mcg/kg/min

* Here is another example for you to work out. Answers are on the bottom of the next page:

  Dobutamine 500mg in 250cc D5W. Pt weight 220lbs.
  1. Start dobutamine at 5mcg/kg/hr
  2. The rate is now 10cc/hr .What is the dosage in mcg/Kg/min?
        (ensure that you are working with the proper units)

Pulmonary Formulas

Pao_2 = Partial pressure of Oxygen. Oxygen dissolved in plasma
Sao_2 = Oxygen saturation. Percent Oxygen bound to hemoglobin.
Cao_2 = Arterial Oxygen content. Total amount of oxygen carried
     in the blood. Pao_2 and Sao_2, reported in ml/100ml or as %

* **Henderson-Hasselbach Equation (blood pH)**
    $pH = pK(6.1) + \log (HCO_3 \text{ mEq/L (Base)} / Paco_2 \text{mmHg} \times .03 \text{ (Acid)})$
* **Partial Pressure of Oxygen in the alveolus (PAo_2, in mmHg)**
    $PAo_2 = PIo_2 - (Paco_2 \times 1.25)$
* **Arterial Oxygen Saturation (Sao_2)**
    $(Hgbo_2 / Hgb + Hgbo_2) \times 100$ Normal: >92%
* **Arterial Oxygen Content (Cao_2)**
    1. Calculate amount of oxygen dissolved in 100 ml of plasma:
       $Pao_2 \times 0.003 = \text{ml } O_2/100 \text{ ml plasma}$
    2. Calculate amount of oxygen bound to hemoglobin:
       $Hgb \times 1.34 \times Sao_2 = \text{ml of } O_2 \text{ bound to Hgb}$
    3. Add results of steps 1 and 2 for CaO_2 in vol. %
Example: Patient has Pao_2 100 mmHg, Sao_2 .95, Hgb 15g%
    1. $100 \times 0.003 = .3 \text{ml } O_2$ in 100 ml plasma
    2. $15 \text{ g}\% \times 1.34 \times .95 = 19.10 \text{ ml } O_2$ bound to Hgb
    3. $0.3 + 19.1 = 19.4 \text{ vol}\% CaO_2$
* **Venous Oxygen Content (Cvo_2)**
  Same as Cao_2 but substitute Svo_2 and Pvo_2 for arterial values (Sao_2, Pao_2)
* **Tissue Oxygen Consumption (Vo_2)**
$(CO \times Cao_2 \times 10) - (CO \times Cvo_2 \times 10)$
       Arterial - Venous   (normal 250ml/min)

(Answer to Dosage Formula problem: Weight = 100Kg
Concentration = 2000mcg/cc. Rate = 15 cc/hr. Dose = 3.3mcg/kg/hr)

Cardiac Formulas

- **Cardiac Output   CO = HR X SV**   (normal 4-8L/min)
- **Cardiac Index   CI=CO/BSA**(body surface area. NML 2.2-4.4L/min/m^2)
- **Stroke Volume SV = (CO/HR) 1000**   (normal 60-70 ml)
- **Mean Arterial Pressure (MAP)**
    (Diastolic x 2) + (Systolic x 1) / 3   (normal 70-100mmHg)
- **Systemic Vascular Resistance (SVR)**
    MAP – RAP (R atrial pressure) / CO = SVR in units (normal 10-18 units)
    Result multiplied by 80 = SVR in dynes/sec/cm^{-5}
    (normal 800-1400 dynes/sec/cm^{-5})
- **Systemic Vascular Resistance Index (SVRI)**
    (MAP-RAP / CI) x 80 (normal SVRI 2000-2400 dynes/sec/cm^{-5}/m^2)
- **Pulmonary Vascular Resistance (PVR)**
    PAP (pulmonary artery pressure). PAWP (Pulmonary artery wedge pressure)
    PAP mean – PAWP / CO = PVR in units (normal 1.2-3.0 units)
    Result multiplied by 80 = PVR in dynes/sec/cm^{-5}
    (normal 100-250 dynes/sec/cm^{-5})
- **Pulmonary Vascular Resistance Index (PVRI)**
    (PAP mean – PAWP / CI) x 80 (normal PVRI 225-315 dynes/sec/cm^{-5}/m^2)
- **Left Cardiac Work Index (LCWI)**
    MAP x CO x 0.0136 = LCW
    LCW/BSA = LCWI (normal 3.4-4.2kg-m/m^2)
- **Left Ventricular Stroke Work Index (LVSWI)**
    MAP x SV x 0.0136 = LVSW
    LVSW/BSA = LVSWI (normal 50-62g-m/m^2)
- **Right Cardiac Work Index (RCWI)**
    PAP mean x CO x 0.0136 = RCW
    RCW/BSA = RCWI (normal 0.54-0.66 kg-m/m^2)
- **Right Ventricular Stroke Work Index (RVSWI)**
    PAP mean x SV x 0.0136 = RVSW
    RVSW/BSA = RVSWI (normal 7.9-9.7 g-m/m^2)

Other Formulas

* **Cerebral Perfusion Pressure (CPP)**
  MAP – ICP (normal 80-100mmHg)
  Normal ICP 0-15mmHg   Severe ↑ICP >20mmHg

* **Estimating Energy Needs**

Step 1 (Harris-Benedict Equations)
♀ = 655 + (9.56 x weight (kg)) + (1.85 x height (cm)) – (4.68 x age (years))
♂ = 66.5 + (13.8 x weight (kg)) + (5 x height (cm)) – (6.76 x age (in years))

Step 2 Multiply result by activity level

Activity Level	Multiply by
Bed rest	1.2
Light	1.3
Moderate	1.4
Strenuous	1.5 or more

Step 3 Multiply step 2 by stressor

Stressor	Multiply by
Fever	1 + 0.13/^{0}C above nml (or 0.07/^{0}F above nml)
Pneumonia	1.2
Major injury	1.3
Severe sepsis	1.5-1.6
Major burns	1.8-2.0

* **Estimating Protein Needs**

Condition	Multiply desirable body weight (kg) by
Healthy individual (elective surgery patient)	0.8-1g protein
Malnourished or catabolic state (sepsis, burns, injury)	1.2-2+g protein

Tenormin (atenolol)

Rate slide rule
- magnifier

HR   standard intervals

cm   magnifier

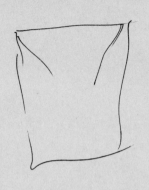

Na | Cl | BUN
K | CO2| Cr \ Glu

WBC > Hgb/Hct < Plt

Resuscitation

Ventricular Fibrillation/Pulseless Ventricular Tachycardia

- CPR until defibrillator available
- Defibrillate up to 3 times if needed @ 200 J, @ 200-300 J and 360 J
- CPR, IV access, and intubate
- Epinephrine 1.0mg IVP q 3-5 min.
- Defibrillate @ 360 J within 30-60 sec.
- Meds:
  - Lidocaine 1.5mg/kg IVP q 3-5min. Total of 3mg/kg then use
  - Bretylium 5mg/kg IVP repeat in 10 min @ 10mg/kg
  - Magnesium sulfate 1-2g IV in torsades de pointes, or hypomagnesemic state, or severe refractory VF
  - Procainamide 30mg/min in refractory VF (max 17mg/kg)
  - Consider sodium bicarbonate 1mEq/kg IV
- Defibrillate @ 360 J, 30-60 sec. (drug-shock, drug-shock)

Asystole

- CPR, IV access and intubate
- Confirm asystole in more than one lead
- Consider possible cause
- Consider immediate transcutaneous pacing (TCP)
- Epinephrine 1.0mg IVP q 3-5 min.
- Atropine 1mg IV q 3-5 min. to a total of 0.04mg/kg or 3mg
- Consider sodium bicarbonate
- Consider termination of efforts

Tachycardia

- If unstable with serious signs and symptoms (if HR>150) cardiovert
- Look at rhythm: Afib/flutter? PSVT? Vtach? Wide complex, uncertain?
  - Atrial fibrillation/Atrial flutter:
    - Consider: Diltiazem, beta-blockers, verapamil, digoxin, procainamide, quinidine, anticoagulants
  - Paroxysmal supraventricular tachycardia:
    - Vagal maneuvers (carotid pressure contraindicated with carotid bruits)
    - Adenosine 6mg rapid IVP over 1-3 sec.
    - Adenosine 12mg rapid IVP over 1-3 sec. (may repeat once after 1-2 min.)
    - Complex width?
      - Narrow: If BP low/unstable then cardiovert. If BP nml or↑ then verapamil 2.5-5mg IV. In 15-30min repeat @ 5-10mg Consider digoxin, beta blockers, diltiazem. Cardiovert
      - Wide: Lidocaine 1-1.5mg/kg IVP. Procainamide 20-30mg/min, max 17mg/kg. Cardiovert
  - Ventricular tachycardia (with a pulse):
    - Lidocaine 1-1.5mg/kg IVP q5-10min.
    - Lidocaine 0.5-0.75mg/kg IVP max 3mg/kg
    - Procainamide 20-30mg/min. max. 17mg/kg
    - Bretylium 5-10mg/kg over 8-10min. max. 30mg/kg over 24hr
    - Cardiovert
  - Wide complex tachycardia of uncertain type:
    - Lidocaine 1-1.5mg/kg IVP q5-10min
    - Lidocaine 0.5-0.75mg/kg IVP max 3mg/kg
    - Adenosine 6mg rapid IVP over 1-3 sec.
    - Adenosine 12mg rapid IVP over 1-3 sec. (may repeat once after 1-2 min.)
    - Procainamide 20-30mg/min. max. 17mg/kg
    - Bretylium 5-10mg/kg over 8-10min. max. 30mg/kg over 24hr
    - Cardiovert

Bradycardia

- Serious signs and symptoms?
  - Yes:
    - Atropine 0.5-1.0mg q3-5min up to 0.04mg/kg or 3mg
    - TCP if available
    - Dopamine 5-20μg/kg/min
    - Epinephrine 2-10μg/min
    - Isoproterenol (use with caution)
    - If 2nd degree heart block type II or 3rd degree heart block then prepare for transvenous pacer. Use TCP as bridge device
  - No:
    - If sinus, juctional, 1st degree heart block or 2nd degree type I then treat only if signs or symptoms, observe
    - If 2nd degree heart block type II or 3rd degree heart block then prepare for transvenous pacer. Use TCP as bridge device

"To me, it's always a good idea to always carry two sacks of something when you walk around. That way, if anybody says, "Hey, can you give me a hand?" you can say, "Sorry, got these sacks."

Jack Handey

Notes:

Nitroprusside converted
to cyanide ions in
bloodstream.

Syringe Compatibility

Locate first drug on left column. Note the appropriate number of second drug and find its location along the top row. Compatibility is found on the grid square where the name of the first drug and the number of the second drug meet

	1	2	3	4	5	6	7	8	9	10	11	12	13	14	15	16	17	18	19
Atropine (1)		C		I	C	C		C	C	C	C	C	C	C	C	C	C	I	
Butorphanol (2) *Stadol*	C			I	C		I	C	C	C	C	C	I	C	C		C	I	C
Codeine (3)				I									I					I	
Diazepam (4) *Valium*	I	I	I		I	I		I	I	I		I	I	I	I		I	I	I
Fentanyl (5)	C	C		I		C		C	C	C		C	I	C	C	C	C	I	
Glycopyrrolate (6) *Robinul*	C			I	C			C	C			C	I	C	C	C	C	I	
Heparin (7)		I		I					I			I			I				
Hydroxyzine (8) *Atarax, Vistaril*	C	C		I	C	C			C	C		C	I	C	I	C	I	C	I
Meperidine (9) *Demerol, Pethadol*	C	C		I	C	C	I	C		C		I	I	C	C	C	C	I	
Metoclopramide (10) *Reglan, Maxolon*	C	C		I	C			C	C			C		C	C	C	C	I	
Midazolam (11) *Versed*	C	C			C	C		C		C		C	I	I	C	I	C		C
Morphine (12)	C	C		I	C	C	I	C	I	C			I	C	C	C	C	I	
Pentobarbital (13) *Nembutal*	C	I	I	I	I	I		I	I	I		I		I	I	I	I	C	
Prochlorperazine (14) *Compazine*	C	C		I	C	C		C	C	C		C	I		C	C	C	I	
Promethazine (15) *Phenergan*	C	C		I	C	C		C	C	C		C	I	C		C	C	I	
Ranitidine (16) *Zantac*	C				C	C		I	C	C	I	C		C	C		C		C
Scopolamine Hbr (17)	C	C		I	C	C		C	C	C		C	I	C	C	C		I	
Secobarbital (18)	I	I	I	I	I	I	I	I	I	I		I	I	I	I		I		I
Thiethylperazine (19) *Torecan*		C	I													C		I	

C = Compatible

Common trade names in *Italics*

I = Incompatible

☐ = No documented information

Cardiovascular Drugs

Antidysrhythmics: Correct abnormal cardiac cycles. Different agents act through different means. Classification system in use: Class I – Class IV.

Class I: Sodium channel blockers. Prolong refractory period by ↓influx of Na ions (further subdivided into class IA, IB, and IC. Agents in these categories include quinidine, procainamide, and lidocaine).

Class II: Beta blockers. Block or compete with endogenous catecholamines for receptor sites (further subdivided into cardioselective –block only beta$_1$- and noncardioselective –block both beta$_1$ and beta$_2$ – Drugs in this category include propranolol, acebutolol, esmolol).

Class III: These drugs prolong duration of action potential (bretylium, amiodarone, sotalol).

Class IV: Calcium channel blockers. ↓influx of Ca at SA and AV nodes thereby ↓ conduction. Also relax coronary smooth muscle and dilate coronary arteries. Verapamil is in this category. Accessory pathways not affected by verapamil therefore should not be used in Wolff-Parkinson-White syndrome.

Adenosine: Not classified in above system. It acts by causing a transient AV block and it is indicated for treatment of supraventricular tachycardias.

Inotropics: Enhance cardiac contractility. Include cardiac glycosides (digitalis and derivatives), sympathomimetics (epinephrine, dopamine, dobutamine, norepinephrine, isoproterenol) and phosphodiesterase inhibitors (Inocor).

Vasodilators: Dilate arteries and veins reducing preload/afterload thus enhancing cardiac output without ↑myocardial Oxygen demands. Various categories including direct smooth muscle relaxants (nitroglycerin, Nipride), Calcium channel blockers (Procardia, verapamil, Cardizem), ACE inhibitors (Capoten, Vasotec), alpha-adrenergic blockers (labetalol –alpha and beta blocker, Regitine) and vasopressors (epinephrine, norepinephrine, Neo-Synephrine).

Characteristics of Selected Cardiac Drugs (adults)

Drug	Indication/Action	Dosage	Major Side Effects
Adenosine	Paroxysmal SVT	6mg rapid IVP, repeat 12mg, follow with IV fluid (NS or D₅W)	Flushing, dyspnea, hypotension
Bretylium	Refractory V Fib.	5mg/kg IV followed by 10mg/kg @15-30min intervals max. 30mg/kg	HTN, tachycardia, PVCs
Captopril (Capoten)	Hypertension. Vasodilator, moderate preload and afterload effects	25-150mg PO bid-tid max 450mg	Hypotension, chronic cough, neutropenia
Dopamine	Dose related: low dosages (1-2µg/kg/min) ↑renal perfusion and urinary output. Moderate dosages (<10µg/kg/min) ↑myocardial contractility and improves CO. High dosages (>10µg/kg/min) vasoconstriction, negation of dopaminergic effects		Tachycardia, HTN, angina, wide QRS. Extravasation: watch for tissue problems, gangrene
Dobutamine	Heart failure	2.5-10µg/kg/min. May increase to 40µg/kg/min. if needed	Anxiety, palpitations, PVCs
Lidocaine	Ventricular ectopy, MI	50-100mg IV bolus then 1-4mg/min infusion	CNS toxicity, convulsions, heart block, respiratory depression
Nitroglycerin	Angina, CHF associated with acute MI	5-300µg/min IV inf. SL.: 1 tab. when pain begins, repeat q5min. until relief. No more than 3 tabs/15min.	Headache, reflex tachycardia, hypotension
Verapamil	SVT	5-10mg IV >2min.10mg in 30min. if needed	Edema, CHF, bradycardia, AV block, dizziness

Thrombolytic Therapy Guide

Thrombolytics act by converting plasminogen to plasmin (plasmin is able to break donwn blood clots). They are used as treatment in an acute MI, as well as to treat DVT, PE, arterial embolism and arterial thrombosis. Agents in this category include urokinase, streptokinase, anistreplase (APSAC), and alteplase (t-PA). Their adult use in treatment of an acute MI is discussed here.

Thrombolytic Therapy Selection Criteria

- Not > 6 hours from onset of chest pain. Less if possible
- Documented ST segment elevation on EKG
- Ischemic chest pain of 30 minutes duration
- Chest pain not responding to sublingual nitroglycerin or nifedipine
- < 76 years old
- No conditions that might cause a predisposition to hemorrhage (recent surgery, recent CVA, coagulation disorders, etc.)
- No active bleeding

Thrombolytic Agents and Management (for use in MI)

	Streptokinase	APSAC	t-PA
Fibrin Selective	No	Semiselective	Yes
Half-life	<20 min (interm.)	105 min (long)	10 (short)
Dose	1.5 MU	30 U over 2-5 min. asap after sx onset	100mg total. 60mg over 1st hr. 20mg over 2nd, 20mg over 3rd hour.
Hypotension	Present	May be present	Not present
Allergic Reaction	Present	Present	Not present
Other Considerations	Monitor: Gullain-Barre syndrome may occur after tx	Do not mix with any other solution or drug	Do not use 150mg or more: IC bleeding may occur

General Considerations: PT, or aPTT <2 x control before starting tx. Monitor clotting times q3-4h during tx. Monitor for S+S of internal bleeding (temp >104, neuro changes, back pain, leg weakness, ↓pulse, hematuria, hematemesis, ecchymosis, epistaxis). Guaiac stools. <u>Monitor cardiac rhythm and non-invasive evidence of reperfusion</u>: Cessation of chest pain, ST back to baseline, early and marked peaking of CK. Monitor for reperfusion arrhythmias

Commonly Used Analgesics in Adults

Acetaminophen (Tylenol) PO 365-650mg q4-6hr (max 4g/d)	**Hydrocodone and acetaminophen** (Vicodin) PO 1-2 tabs q4-6hr
Acetaminophen with codeine PO15-60mg q4-6hr	**Ibuprofen** (Advil, Motrin, Nuprin) 200-800mg/dose tid-qid
Chloral hydrate (Aquachloral) 250mg tid anxiety, 500-1000mg qhs for insomnia (max 2g/d)	**Mefenamic acid** (Ponstel) 500mg then 250mg q4-6hr not to exceed 1 week
Codeine 10-20mg/dose q4-6hr (max 120mg/qd)	**Meperidine** (Demerol) PO/SC/IM 50-150 mgq3-4hr prn. Preop: IM/SC 50-100mg q30-90min. Reduce doses if IV
Cyclobenzaprine (Flexeril) 20-40mg/d divided q6-12h (max 60mg/d)	**Naproxen** (Naprosyn) Rheumatoid arthritis: 500-1000mg/d; analgesia: 250mg q6-8hr (max 1250 mg/d)
Fentanyl Anesthetic:IV 0.05-0.1mg q2-3min prn. Preop:IM 0.05-0.1mg q30-60min. Postop:IM 0.05-0.1mg q1-2hr prn	**Oxycodone** (Percocet, Roxicet) PO 5mg q4-6hr or 10mg tid or qid prn

General Nursing Implications: Assess renal, liver and blood studies. Evaluate therapeutic effect; assess objectively pain relief. Advise client to avoid driving and other hazardous activity, monitor for CNS depression and advise of potential for physical dependence (narcotics, hypnotics). Do not use with alcohol. Watch out for interactions and contraindications with MAO inhibitors, tricyclic antidepressants, CNS depressants and anti-coagulants.

Treatment for Narcotic Overdose: Naloxone (Narcan) 0.2-0.8mg IV, O_2, IV fluids, vasopressors.

Commonly Used Respiratory Drugs in Adults

Metaproterenol (Alupent) Long-acting bronchodilator. MDI 2-3 puffs q3-4hr not >12 puffs/day.	**Atropine** Bronchodilation and drying up secretions. Nebulizer: 0.05mg/kg diluted in NS tid-qid
Aminophylline For Tx of bronchospasms. Titrate dosage to maintain therapeutic serum level 10-20µg/ml. Toxic >20µg/ml. Not compatible in syringe with any drugs	**Albuterol** (Proventil, Ventolin) For Bronchospasm: MDI 1-2 puffs q4-6hr. PO 2-4mg tid-qid, not to exceed 8mg
Isoetharine (Bronkosol) Bronchodilator with few cardiac side effects. INH 3-7 puffs undiluted. IPPB 0.5ml diluted 1:3 with NS	**Epinephrine** For asthma: INH 1-2 puffs of 1:1000 or 2.25% racemic q15min
Terbutaline (Brethine) MDI 2 puffs q1min. then q4-6h. IV dilute 5mg/1L D₅W inf. To run 5µg/min. may ↑5µg q10min, titrate to response. After ½ - 1hr, taper dose by 5µg. Switch to PO as soon as possible. PO 2.5-5mg q8h	**Isoproterenol** (Isuprel) Potent bronchodilator. SL 10-20mg q6-8hr. MDI 1 puff, may repeat in 2-5min. Maintenance 1-2 puffs 4-6X/day. IV 10-20µg during anesthesia (monitor EKG)
Acetylcysteine (Mucomyst) As mucolytic agent: administer after proper respiratory hygene. Usually given with bronchodilator 1-2ml (10-20% sol) q1-4hr prn or 3-5ml (20%) or 6-10 ml (10%) tid or qid (also used in Acetaminophen poisoning)	**Zafirlukast** (Accolate) Fairly new, antagonizes the contractile action of leukotrines thereby inhibiting bronchoconstriction. For prophylaxis and chronic treatment of asthma. PO 20mg bid 1hr ac or 2 hr pc (not a beta adrenergic agonist)

General Nursing Implications: Bronchodilators above mostly stimulate beta receptors responsible for bronchial dilation *and* CNS and cardiac stimulation. Therefore, palpitations and tachycardia are usual side effects. Watch out for more severe cardiac effects (dysrhythmias, arrest). Due to CNS stimulation, give at least 2hr before hs. Do not use with other sympathomimetics or MAO inhibitors. Potentiated by tricyclic antidepressants, antihistamines and levothyroxine.

Insulin Preparations

Type of Insulin	Time of onset (hr)	Peak of action (hr)	Duration of action (hr)	Appearance
Rapid acting				
Insulin lispro (Humalog)	15 min	40-60 min	46 min half-life	Clear
Regular	<1	2-4	4-6	Clear
Crystalline zinc	<1	2-4	5-8	Clear
Semilente	1-2	3-10	10-16	Cloudy
Intermediate				
NPH	1-2	4-12	18-24	Cloudy
Globin zinc	2-4	6-10	12-18	Clear
Lente	1-3	6-15	18-24	Cloudy
Slow acting				
Protamine zinc	4-8	14-24	36+	Cloudy
Ultralente	4-8	10-30	28-36	Cloudy

"The best and most beautiful things in the world cannot be seen or even touched. They must be felt within the heart."

Helen Keller

References

American Heart Association: *Handbook of emergency cardiovascular care for healthcare providers,* Dallas, 1997, American Heart Association.

Fonarow, Gregg, C.: *UCLA clinical practice guideline: Cardiac troponin I assay diagnostic module,* 1996. Available: http://www.cost-quality.com/2%2C3art.html

Jarvis, Carolyn: *Physical examination and health assessment,* ed 2, Philadelphia, 1996, WB Saunders.

Glanze, D. Walter, managing editor: *Mosby's medical, nursing & allied health dictionary,* ed 3, St. Louis, 1990, Mosby.

Hall, B. Jesse; Schmidt G. & Wood L.: *Principles of critical care, companion handbook,* New York, 1993, McGraw-Hill.

LeFever, Joyce Kee: *Laboratory and diagnostic tests with nursing implications,* ed 5, Stamford, 1999, Appleton & Lange.

Lanros, E. Nedell & Janet M. Barber: *Emergency Nursing,* ed 4, Stamford, 1997, Appleton & Lange.

Marieb, N. Elaine, *Human anatomy and physiology,* Redwood City, 1989, Benjamin Cummings.

Skidmore-Roth, Linda: *Mosby's 1999 nursing drug reference,* St. Louis, 1999, Mosby.

Stilltwell, B. Susan: *Quick critical care reference,* St. Louis, 1994, Mosby

Swartz, H. Mark: *Textbook of physical diagnosis: history and examination,* ed 2, Philadelphia, 1994, WB Saunders.

Thelan, A. Lynne et al: *Critical care nursing: diagnosis and management,* ed 2, St. Louis, 1994, Mosby.